LYNEAH MARKS

The Truth About Stress

The Truth Will Set you FREE

First published by Body, Soul & Angels Publishing 2024

Copyright © 2024 by Lyneah Marks

All rights reserved. No part of this publication may be reproduced, stored or transmitted in any form or by any means, electronic, mechanical, photocopying, recording, scanning, or otherwise without written permission from the publisher. It is illegal to copy this book, post it to a website, or distribute it by any other means without permission.

Lyneah Marks asserts the moral right to be identified as the author of this work.

Lyneah Marks has no responsibility for the persistence or accuracy of URLs for external or third-party Internet Websites referred to in this publication and does not guarantee that any content on such Websites is, or will remain, accurate or appropriate.

Designations used by companies to distinguish their products are often claimed as trademarks. All brand names and product names used in this book and on its cover are trade names, service marks, trademarks and registered trademarks of their respective owners. The publishers and the book are not associated with any product or vendor mentioned in this book. None of the companies referenced within the book have endorsed the book.

Second edition

ISBN: 978-0-9889827-6 5

This book was professionally typeset on Reedsy.
Find out more at reedsy.com

To all who pioneered this path and those who have followed it pushing the grass down so we could more easily follow.

Contents

Acknowledgement		ii
Introduction		1
1	The Truth About Stress	3
2	What to do?	11
3	The Five Basic Exercises: Overview	15
4	Concentration	19
5	Controlling the Will	25
6	Equanimity	28
7	Positivity	34
8	Open Mindedness	37
9	Cycling all Five Basic Exercises	41
10	Rückshau – Looking Back Exercise	44
11	Physical and Energetic Helpers	47
12	Conclusion and Continuance	53
13	Bonus Meditation	57
14	Journal	60
15	Notes/Observations	65
About the Author		68
Also by Lyneah Marks		69

Acknowledgement

Gratitude to AIA Publishing for pushing this book out in a shorter time than I thought possible (5 days start to finish without AI), to my husband and friends who have supported and encouraged me, to those who trigger me and thereby encourage me to grow.

Introduction

The TRUTH About

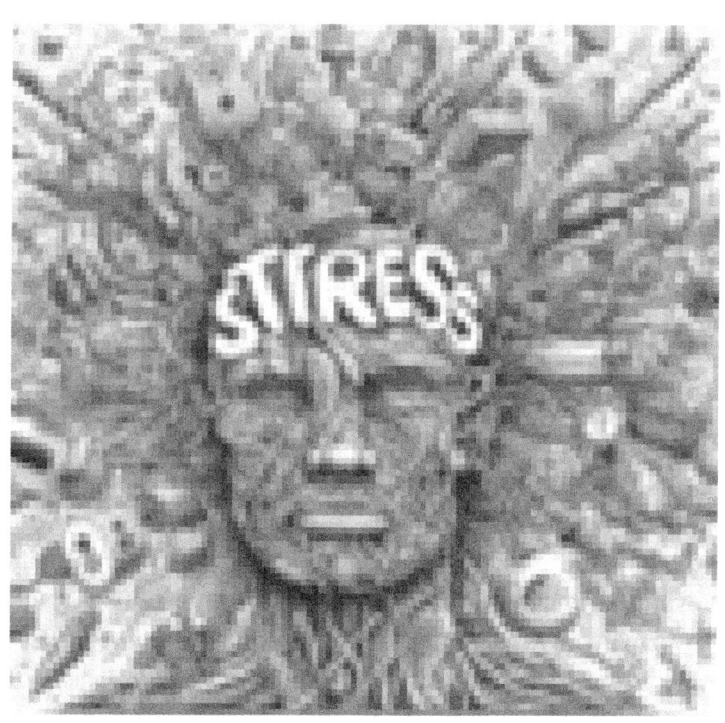

THE TRUTH WILL SET YOU FREE

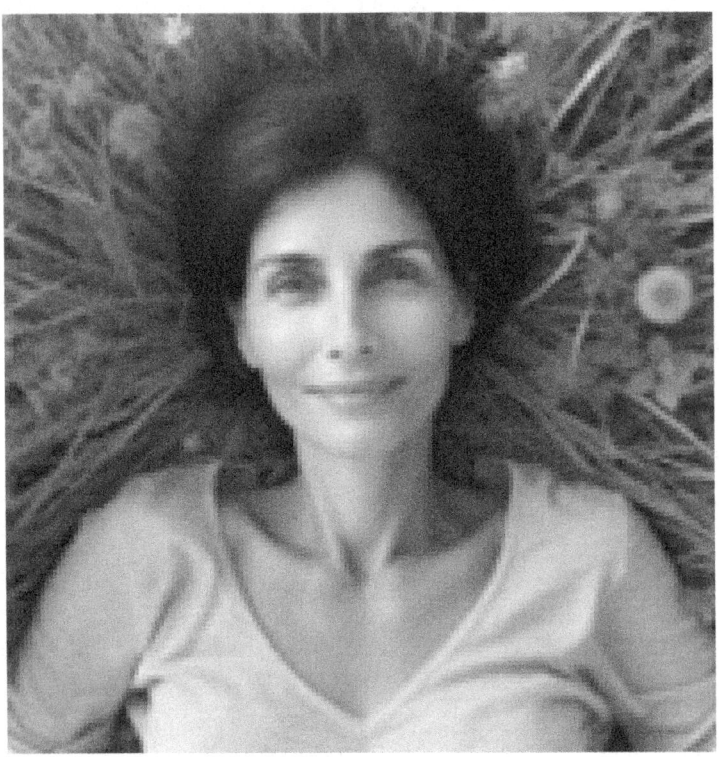

by Lyneah Marks

This book is the result of many years of teaching energy work which led me to teaching the exercises that I have used to build my intuition over the years. This is a condensation of what I cover in Improve Your Intuition Webinar and can help you reduce your stress levels dramatically. Doing the exercises brings great results. I hope you enjoy the process.

1

The Truth About Stress

CHAPTER ONE: THE TRUTH ABOUT STRESS

STRESS CONTRIBUTES TO DIS-EASE

Increasingly more doctors are recognizing stress as a major factor in illness, affecting nearly every aspect of health. Here's what some experts have to say:

- **Henry Ford Health**: *"Stress is known to increase the risk for nearly every disease state, including heart disease, high blood pressure, and a weakened immune system. Chronic stress, if not managed, can lead to serious, even life-threatening diseases."* [1].

- **BMC Health Services Research**: *"Physicians acknowledge the impact of stress on their well-being, with workplace stressors threatening their mental health. Coping strategies and* *resilience are essential to manage these stressors."* [2].

- **HelpGuide.org**: *"Chronic stress disrupts nearly every system in the body, increasing the risk of heart attack, stroke, and mental health problems like anxiety and depression."* [3].

- **Columbia Doctors**: *"Research indicates that chronic stress is associated with health issues such as muscle tension, digestive problems, headaches, weight gain or loss, trouble sleeping, heart disease, susceptibility to cancer, high blood pressure, and stroke."* [4].

We can probably agree that stress is at least a major factor in health but what is stress?

Physiologically we know it is a cascade of substances starting with the adrenals producing cortisol and adrenaline, often referred to as the adrenal complex. These substances stimulate inflammation and inflammation is at the root of many dis-eases. That will do for our purposes. But what causes the adrenals to jump into action?

TYPES OF STRESS:

Sometimes it is something innate like a bomb going off or a loud thunderclap. But what about your boss telling you your report needs more work. Is this stress? Or a person confronting you on an issue at home? Or getting everything ready to do your taxes.

There are at least three types of stress:

INNATE – the kind of life-threatening response to a dinosaur chasing you. This happens if you are confronted with someone with a gun or knife. Well trained warriors even know how to not respond stressfully in such a situation. Grasshopper of Kung Fu fame learns to be calm in the most threatening of circumstances and learns that stepping out of stress helps him stay focused and able to respond – "response able". So even innate stress can be overcome and/or used to your advantage with adequate training.

LEARNED – you saw your mother or father stress before a holiday so you learn to be stressed before holidays. What is learned can be unlearned and we'll be talking about how.

CREATED – you see your boss as a tyrant and you fear for your job. You've created a situation where you are in debt and require your income to survive. You have put yourself in a position where you must work, so you are willing to compromise yourself for your paycheck. You choose to respond stressfully to any situation that might slightly threaten your job. You fear what people think about you, so you stress over what to say and do. In many situations stress is created. Stress is a reaction to things that are not innate stress triggers.

THE TRUTH ABOUT STRESS:

Do you believe the truth can set you free? Have you experienced this in your life? I hope so.

Let's assume the truth can set you free for now.
Well, listen to the following TRUTH...take a deep breath, exhale then read:

STRESS IS NOT WHAT COMES TOWARD YOU,

STRESS IS HOW YOU REACT TO WHAT COMES TOWARD YOU.

Let this in. Imagine feeling you had control over your responses. What would that be like? **Feel** what it would be like if you had total control over whether to respond stressfully or not. Just imagine your world. Imagine yourself. Imagine feeling in control. Take some time to do this before reading more. If this is difficult to imagine, you may come to just the right place.

Most of the time stress is not innate – there are few 'dinosaurs' in our lives - but we have learned to respond stressfully and this type of stress can be unlearned with awareness and effort.

Two people in two different offices have the same situation. The boss is on the rampage and wants an extensive list of things done.

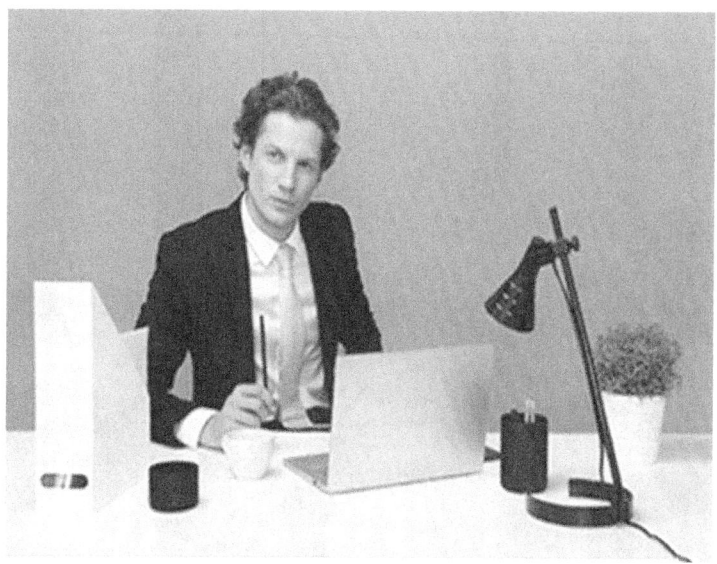

Moose Photos

Person #1, Joe, sits at his office desk worrying over some bills he's not sure how to pay. His boss crashes in yelling about some tasks that needed to be done yesterday. He flares with adrenaline and cortisol soaring though his system putting him into a high state of stressed alert. Interesting, it only takes 17 minutes (average resting rate) for blood to reach all parts of our bodies meaning within 17 minutes the stress factors have stimulated every cell in your body likely raising your blood pressure and your pulse.

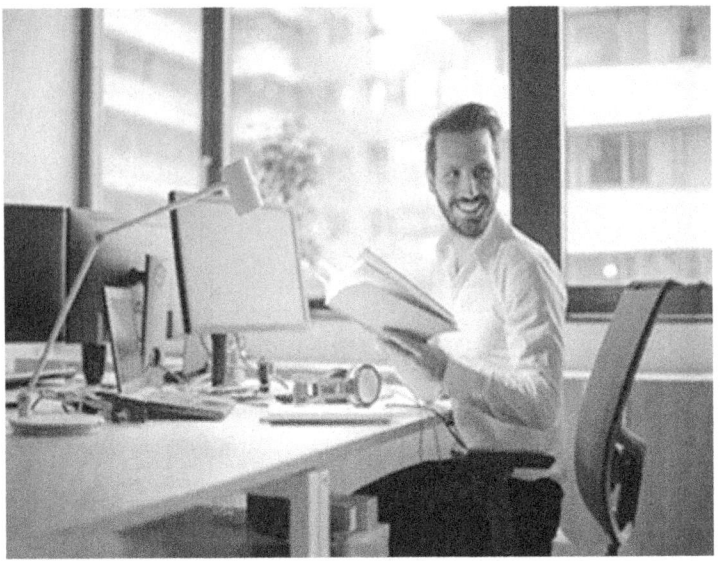

Andrea Piacquadio Photo

Person #2, Jerry, sits at his desk after a morning stretch, a 20-minute walk and a 5-minute concentration exercise which centered and aligned him. The same boss crashes in loudly demanding some work be done. Jerry CHOOSES to continue to be calm and imagines a cascading beautiful waterfall behind the boss. His boss softens a little (power of entrainment see below). Jerry continues deep breathing, one of the things that turns the adrenal complex off. He smiles at the boss sending a calm energetic his way continuing to imagine the waterfall behind his boss. The boss calms a little more (through the power of entrainment explained below) looking a little confused. Jerry repeats what the boss has just asked for, letting him know he's been heard and when the boss nods, Jerry assures him he'll get right on it. Satisfied, the boss leaves with Jerry already starting on the files. Later Jerry learns that the boss' daughter was hospitalized the night before and he is overwhelmed with worry (also a choice).

ENTRAINMENT: This is a basic physics principle which explains interactions between different energies. Two similar energies magnify each other. In the first case person #1, Joe, increased the boss's stress by responding in like kind. Similar frequencies will amplify each other. The result being that both became more stressed. With dissimilar frequencies, the strongest will affect the lesser or weaker volume frequency. Jerry, person #2, has calmed the boss to some extent because he had a strong relaxed energy to start and made a conscious decision to continue to create a peaceful energetic despite the boss' mood. His stronger calm brought the boss into a calmer frequency. Sometimes people leave because they don't want to be calmed and if unaware of what is going on, might be a bit confused or disoriented. Entrainment is a little more complex as a physics principle but for our purposes this explanation is adequate.

Have you ever been at a party that is going well with everyone having a good time and someone comes in who is having a really bad time? Everyone in the room is brought 'down'. That's an example of entrainment. The Dali Lama has spent his life learning to project a strong frequency of peace even in difficult circumstances. If he were at the party, his energy would most likely have been the stronger, the newcomer would have been affected by his strong peaceful energy and calmed down.

Now you know the truth that stress can cause major physical distress and that most stress does not need to be created. The majority of stress is learned and created rather than being innate and even innate stress can be managed with appropriate intention and discipline. In the next chapter we'll talk about what it takes to change our outlook and lower our stress levels.

1. *Stress: 6 things Your doctor Wants you to know.* (n.d.). Henry Ford Health - Detroit, MI. https://www.henryford.com/blog/2016/04/stress-6-things-doctor-wants-you-to-know
2. O'Dowd, E., O'Connor, P., Lydon, S., Mongan, O., Connolly, F., Diskin, C., McLoughlin, A., Rabbitt, L., McVicker, L., Reid-McDermott, B., & Byrne, D. (2018). Stress, coping, and psychological resilience among physicians. *BMC Health Services Research*, *18*(1). https://doi.org/10.1186/s12913-018-3541-8
3. Smith, M., MA. (2024, February 5). *Stress Symptoms, Signs, and causes.* HelpGuide.org. https://www.helpguide.org/articles/stress/stress-symptoms-signs-and-causes.htm
4. *Chronic stress can hurt your overall health.* (2023, July 27). ColumbiaDoctors. https://www.columbiadoctors.org/news/chronic-stress-can-hurt-your-overall-health

2

What to do?

CHAPTER 2: What to do?

The first step is **awareness**, which you have come to in the first chapter if not before you bought this book. You now know that stress is mostly your reaction and you can learn to control it given awareness, intention, exercises and practice.

The second step is your intention to change your life habits around stress. That sounds easy, but it is a serious step. When you strongly set your intention, energies align to help you reach your goal. It's why this step is so important. **WRITE** your intention. Don't skip this step. Writing it makes it more real. You magnetize yourself to draw to you what you need to achieve your goal. This said, take a moment now to set your intention. Write it down. At the end of this book, you will find journal pages for you to document your progress and the first page is reserved for you to write your intention. [LM1] Think about it. It might be something like this:

"I fully intend to change the habit of stress in my life. I intend to draw to me the resources I need to fully embrace this intention."

"I commit to myself to learn ways to reduce stress in my life."

"On this day the _____ of _____, 20___ I formally state that it is my intention to change the habits I learned from my family and friends regarding stress."

"I promise me to take this seriously. I intend to change my life for the better starting now. I will reduce creating stress."

It would be good to dedicate a small journal to this project. Write your intention in your journal so you can review it later.

Write it.

Sign it.

Think of it as a contract with yourself.

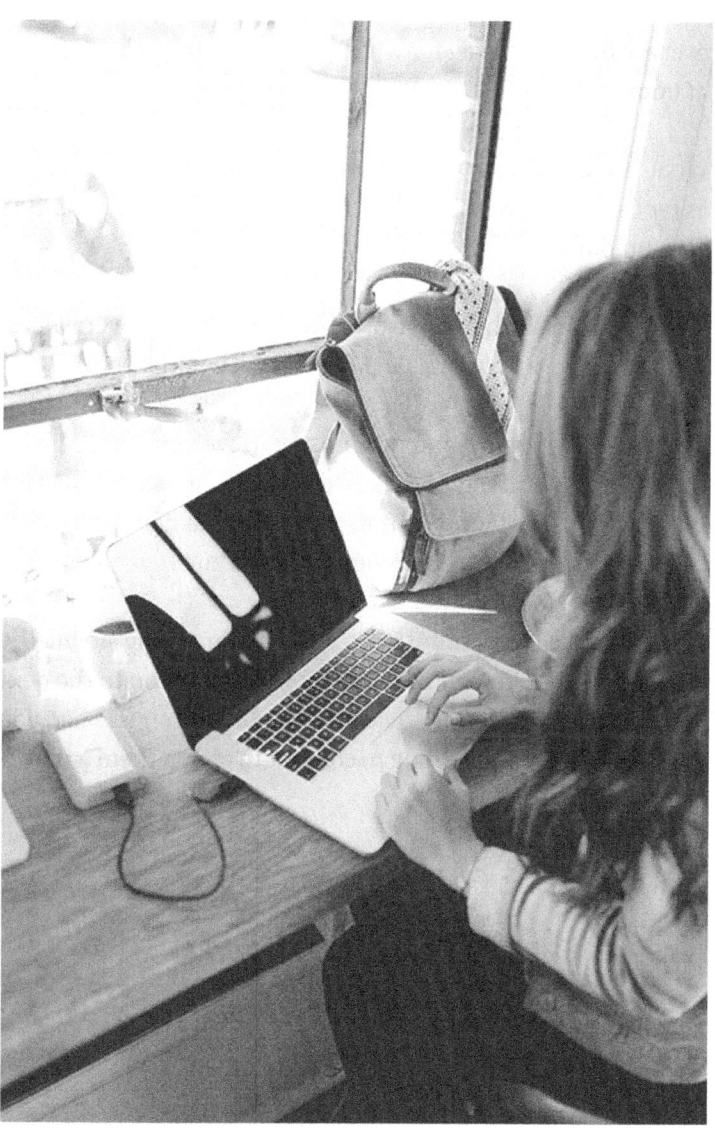

Now, take a moment and rate your general level of stress in your life now. Give it a number between 1 and 100%. Choose an average or enter a level for when you are at work, when you are at home, with family etc. Enter this in your journal.

What percent of your time do you feel stressed? If you want to enter different levels for different circumstances do. Enter this in your journal.

Then think about the degree of stress. What is your overall level of stress? Use a 1 – 100 scale. Enter this in your journal.

Have you filled in the intention page? Have you entered your stress levels? You might make a chart of your stress levels for different circumstances. If not, go and do that now. You owe it to yourself. Then come back here and continue.

Now that you've committed to doing something about the stressful habits in your life, you are ready to go on to the next chapter where we'll introduce the Five Basic Exercises and you can decide if you are willing to commit to giving them a try.

3

The Five Basic Exercises: Overview

The Five Basic Exercises were developed by Dr. Rudolph Steiner over one hundred years ago and millions of people have used them with success. All the quotes in the descriptions of these exercises come out of Dr. Steiner's work.

The Five Basic Exercises are simple but that's not to say easy. They take some time and concentration. Lifting 3 lb. hand weights is relatively easy and if you do it regularly it works. If you don't use them, they won't work. Reading about these exercises is just the beginning. You need to do them to receive the benefits. You will likely find that for the time invested you will receive a great return. They may not look like it on the surface but they are great stress reducers. Over time using them will greatly reduce the level and percentage of time you spend creating stress.

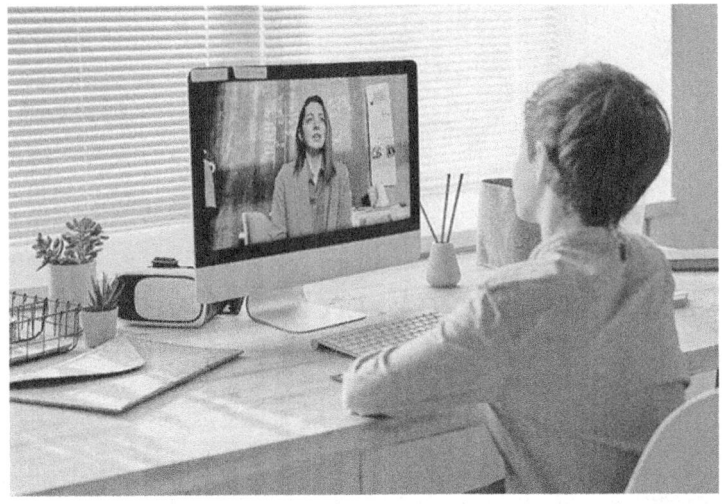

The Five Basic Exercises are great meditations for beginners and advanced individuals alike. They are considered safe even for a novice if you observe Dr. Steiner's two items quoted later in this chapter.

These exercises build organs of perception. It's like going to the gym; if you go and do the work, you build your muscles. In this case the 'muscles' you are building are not something you will see obviously in the mirror. You are more likely to realize one day that you have a different outlook on life and that has made an impact on your comfort level in life and reduced your stress.

I have attended study groups, practiced and then taught classes based on these 5 basic exercises. I have added to them as experience (mine and my students') has shown the need for additional steps. As I already mentioned, the credit for the basics goes to Dr Steiner and the many people over the past more than 100 years who have energized these exercises with goodwill. They have given them a life of their own. You can do these exercises on your own with success and you can join a class or group. You may find accelerated progress when in a well-facilitated group. If you are interested, see the end of this book for an invitation and some testimonials from those who have attended. There you will find instructions for how to put yourself on a mailing list to receive information about a Webinar you can join. The Webinar takes the ideas of this book and puts them into practice in a supportive community where you can have your questions discussed, share your observations and receive encouragement. Over 36 years of practice, every time I lead a class, I do them again and each time I receive added benefits.

A major purpose of these exercises is to gain control of the mind, feelings and impulses of the faculty of will. What is the force that reminds you to do things? Where does that come from? Which thoughts are self-generated and which ones come from outside? How do I know the difference and what's the faculty that knows? These are the 'muscles' we are working on with these exercises. Ponder these questions as you work through them.

The first test comes in devoting at least five minutes of practice each day, preferably at the same time (of your choice), for one week before taking up the next exercise. Dr. Steiner recommended you do 7 consecutive days and if a day is missed, begin again until the seven-day stretch is continuous. This develops several faculties ('muscles') including strength of will. Then move on to the second exercise for a week and the third, fourth and fifth for a week each. As you master the sequence, you might try doing each exercise for two weeks and later increase until you are doing one exercise per month over five months.

In the beginning you probably need to devote 15 minutes daily to the practice. This will give you time to get yourself settled in, make some observations, do the 5-minute exercise and make a few notes. It is most powerful when performed at the same time daily, however, it is better to do it at a different time than to skip it.

Dr. Steiner in *Knowledge of Higher Worlds'*[1] said these exercises comprise a safe path if you observe two things: first, your motives must be other than self-centered. You must be doing this for higher reasons than just your personal gain. For example, wanting to make the world a better place qualifies. Second, you must have great patience with yourself. You must not push yourself. This may sound easy, but you will likely experience challenges in providing yourself with the time to grow on this journey. Know that if you are doing the exercises, you are gaining skills, toning 'muscles'. You don't see results in the gym after one session, so know you need to persist to see the improvements. One day you'll realize, oh, I did that in a new way, or I responded in a new way. You will find yourself reacting more calmly a little at a time. In the next Chapter we'll cover the basics of Exercise 1: Concentration.

[1] Rudolph Steiner, How to Know Higher Worlds: A Modern Path of Initiation, many editions. Rudolph Steiner Knowledge of Higher Worlds, ISBN: 088010046X , Steiner Books, 1983

4

Concentration

Basic Exercise 1: Concentration

This exercise requires a **dedicated 5-minute period** of concentration, preferably at the same time each day. If you cannot manage that, my experience and that of my students' have shown that it will benefit you if you do it daily even if at different times. You'll need a few minutes of preparation and a few minutes to jot down your experience highlights, so set aside 15 minutes. As you go along, the time requirement will reduce.

Choose a simple object, such as a pencil. Decide if it is yellow, has a number, has an eraser, whether it is sharp or not, whether the eraser is chewed or new. This is often referred to as "The Pencil Exercise" for many have chosen a simple pencil as their target of focus. You don't have to choose a pencil but choose something plain that does not remind you of eating or something that might distract your ability to focus. It needs to be a stationary object and the goal is to keep it still and the same day after day.

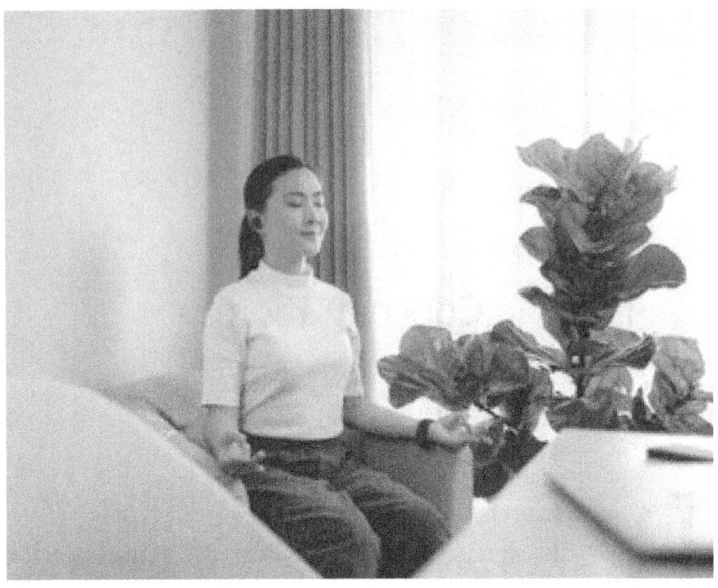

It is not intended to be an exciting exercise. It is intended to further your ability to concentrate in a focused way despite the boredom. 36 years later I am still using the exact same pencil when I do this exercise. The goal is to exclude every other thought and feeling, holding the object still in your mind.

If it is difficult for you to visualize the object, you can try holding it in front of you, staring at it and holding the after image. If this remains problematic, you can take a simple phrase like, "Rain freshens the air," and maintain it for 5 minutes instead of the object. Keep watch for ideas trying to break in on your train of thought.

Pick a time and a place to do your meditation. Make it as clean and simple as possible.

CONCENTRATION

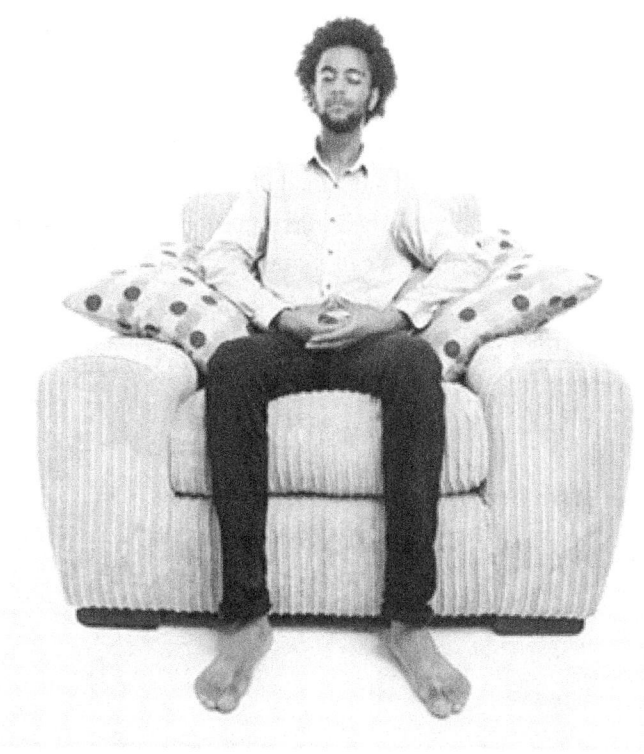

When you sit down to get quiet, the first stage is often a list of things you need to do. Use the "TO DO" page after the Intention page at the back of this book or in a separate journal to jot down things that need to be done. Once written, your mind will be at ease when you have heard what it is telling you and it is more likely to get quiet. Allow a few minutes for this to complete. Resisting those thoughts usually just causes persistence, so listen, jot and release.

Our world is full of images that flash quickly and change

frequently. We are so accustomed to distractions and adjusting to interruptions and five full minutes on just one thing may be a simple task but not necessarily an easy one. If you have young children or pets it might be especially challenging. You might need to set a time when it is most likely they will give you peace and set your intention not to be interrupted. Of course, turn off your phone. Rarely is there a call that won't wait 5 minutes.

The next thing that may surface is something from a movie or interaction that is unresolved. See if you can resolve it in your mind/feelings or jot it down as a thing to take are of later with your to do list.

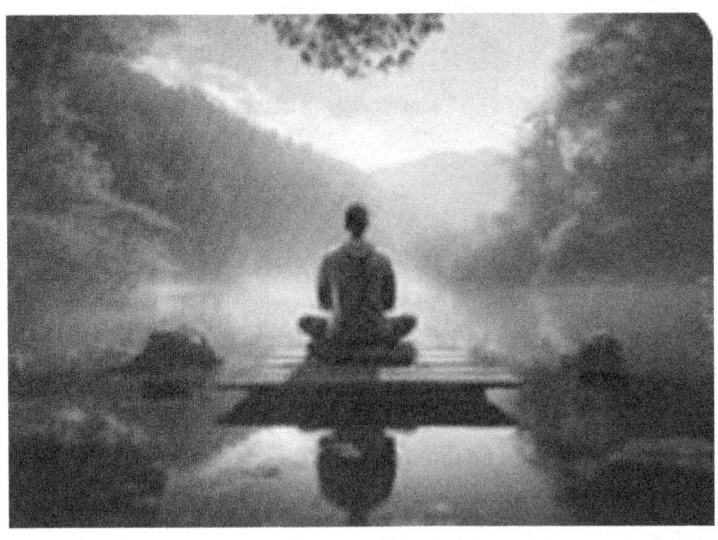

Outside can seem a lovely place to do this work, but there are many distractions including weather, bugs and animals. Once you have mastered this exercise, you might try it in places with distractions to improve your focus, but that will come later. After doing it for several years, I started doing it in Grand Central Station (really - the one in New York City) and airports to strengthen my abilities. In the beginning, use an indoor quiet place.

You can set a timer to let you know when the five minutes are up. It will become easier and easier as you practice, especially if you are able to do it at the same time daily. I like to use an hourglass because it does not make noise to distract you. When you get the hang of 5 minutes you won't even need that. Generally, people find they enjoy the time so much that 5 minutes is not enough. If you must be somewhere else by a certain time, of course, you can use an alarm. You are setting a habit your mind will recognize. It is ok to use a timer during the meditation, but it is not recommended to set an alarm to remind you when to do the meditation. Remembering and being mindful is part of the work to be done here. You can put it in your calendar as an item without reminders, notifications, or alarms.

You may even find this becomes one of your favorite times of the day! I like starting my day with this exercise.

After your 5 minutes, jot down brief notes in your journal. What was special about your experience today? How did it differ from the previous times? Make note of the kinds of thoughts which were not your object or phrase and note where they came from (up, down, side, etc.). Were they created by your mind or did they seem to come from outside you? Just note and notice if there are patterns over time.

This exercise should be continued throughout this experience in tandem with the following exercises. Stay with your object for a minimum of the first week or until you've completed 7 consecutive days. Then you have options: stay with the object/phrase for 5 minutes a day or contemplate the exercise you are working on after you move on to 2, 3, 4 and 5.

For example: While practicing Open-Mindedness you could contemplate:

"What does open-mindedness really mean?"

"How does this change my life for the better?"

"Does it affect my creativity?"

Most people find one of the exercises more difficult than others. If you have one that's a challenge, you might contemplate.

"Why is this particular exercise so difficult for me?"

"What do I need to do to master this exercise?"

The insights you achieve might help you modify something to make it easier. Start your exercise and read on to see what next week's exercise will be.

5

Controlling the Will

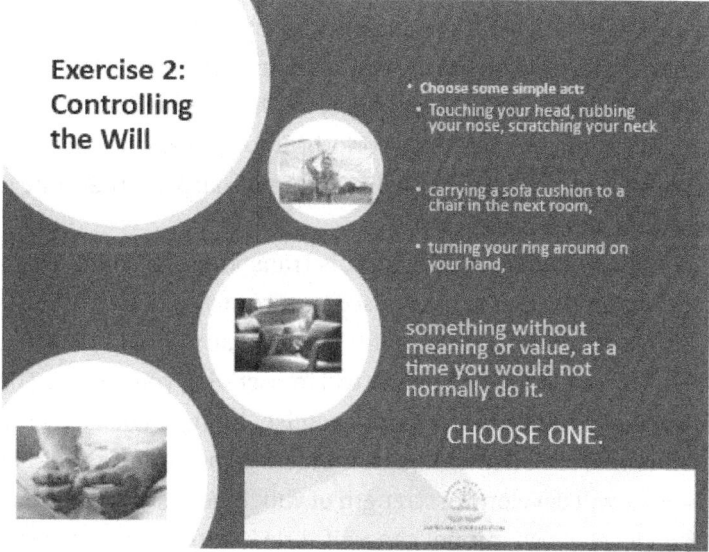

Basic Exercise 2: **Controlling the Will.** Choose some simple act you would not ordinarily do at the time of day you determine, such as carrying a sofa cushion to a chair in the next room, turning your ring around on your hand, rubbing your nose or pulling your ear.

It needs to be something without meaning or value, merely arbitrary. NO ALARMS OR ELETRONIC REMINDERS ALLOWED. You are exercising a 'muscle' that releases an impulse deep inside you that prods you to remember what you have chosen to do at the chosen time. DO IT, daily at the same time. This way you are learning to obey your own commands, training your will forces. The more trivial the action the more difficult it is to arouse the will to do it the more powerful the results. Daily at the same time (that's the goal, it can take some time to get there if this exercise is a challenge for you).

In my life, this one is especially challenging. My schedule varies daily and little in my life is regular, so I have picked first thing in the morning as my time and on other occasions I have picked doing it while brushing my teeth. I have tried noon and 10 am and 10 pm. See what works best for you and as you cycle through this exercise; try a different approach another time if the first was not successful.

I like to have something that is transportable, something I always have with me. I have used turning my ring, brushing my nose and stretching with greater success than things like moving the sofa cushion. Your lifestyle will impact what you choose. The choice is not the object of this exercise. Doing it at exactly the same time each day without reminders is the purpose and that is what will develop the strength of will 'muscles. This exercise also develops your inner sense of time – another nonphysical 'muscle'. This is your second week.

Do you notice any difference in your stress level yet? Make note of changes you observe this week.

"An awakening experience. This class gives you tools that you can

continue to use in everyday life to help strengthen your abilities. I highly recommend anyone wanting to be more in tune with their higher selves and their happiness to take this class."
Shannon Trudeau, LMBT, North Carolina

6

Equanimity

Basic Exercise 3: Equanimity
Here we try to avoid swinging between sympathy and antipathy toward what comes to us from outside. Instead, we try to maintain a balance between the two extremes. We consciously pay attention to our reactions and notice what triggers us to sway from one side to the other.

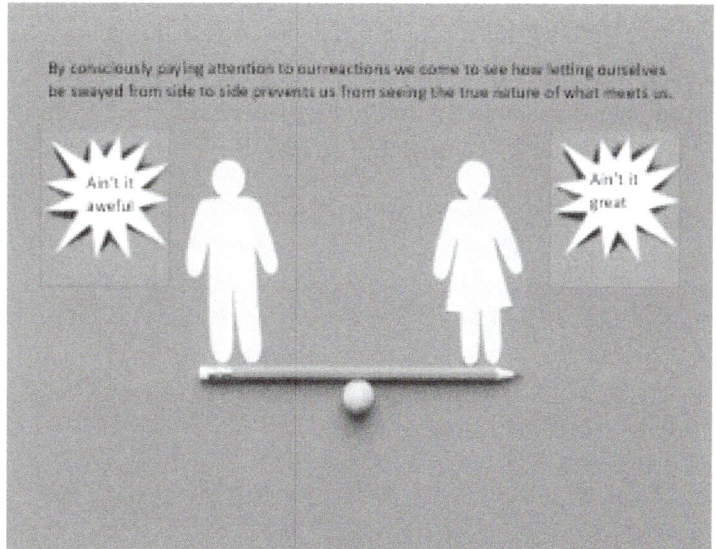

This swaying to either side is coming out of our past experiences and prevents us from seeing the true nature of what meets us. It is survival oriented to be able to generalize from past experience, it increases our probability of survival. However, as we become more receptive to what is actually around us, we can choose our reactions more appropriately. It is often beneficial to avoid extreme expressions of, for instance, elation and sorrow; the one tending to carry us out or ourselves, the other plunging us into despair. This exercise is to help us become capable of maintaining an equable mood, so no sudden situation leads to an outburst of anger or catches us up in anxiety and fear. How often have we judged something bad and reacted with negative emotions, only to find later it was one of the best things that had ever happened?

"Equanimity is important as you progress in your spiritual development for with greater abilities come greater responsibilities. Life

may have already taught you much in this respect, the abilities you gain by your own effort count highly in helping you to move forward in our own development in controlling your world."
Rudolph Steiner

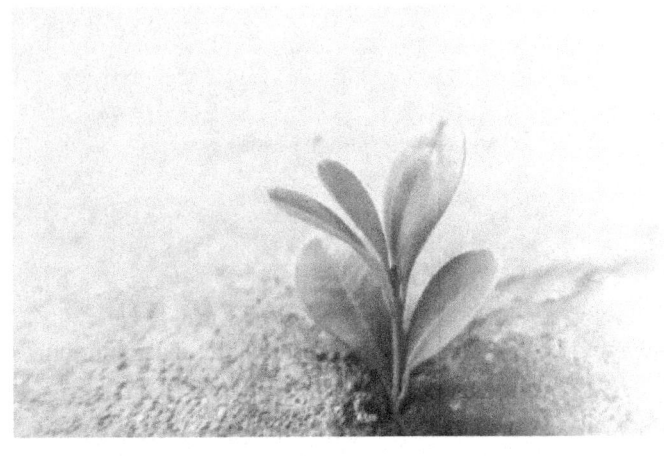

This is not to flatten the spectrum of colors. This exercise is to embrace the fullness of life's experiences and open us up to new ways of being and acting.

"... opening your mind to a kind of inner richness, combined with a transcendence that enables you to very rapidly dissolve the limiting conditioning of the past, not because you are denying it exists but because you have seen so far beyond, you have seen all of the choices for where your conscious awareness can reside, you have seen yourself become entangled with a puzzle, not a problem, a puzzle and all these puzzles are orchestrated. Nothing here in your life is random...do not run from the challenges that life presents you with. You can ask yourself is this roadblock asking me to go in

another direction? What is this life asking me, to get my wrecking ball to clear out a new pathway, so many options available to you...break fixation on experiencing self in any particular way, in recognition that every moment can be new..." [1]

It was also pointed out that previously the Buddhist approach was one of flattening the experiences to make them devoid of emotion. This exercise is not to eliminate emotion, but to consider emotions in a new way. Looking at how you have responded in the past and considering a new way of responding, a new way of being.

One of my favorite Chinese tales might be of help here. The Old Man had a horse which ran away and the neighbors said,

"How sad, how bad. We are so sorry for your misfortune."

He looked at them, grateful for their concern, nodded and said,

"We'll see. We'll see."

The neighbors left shaking their heads.

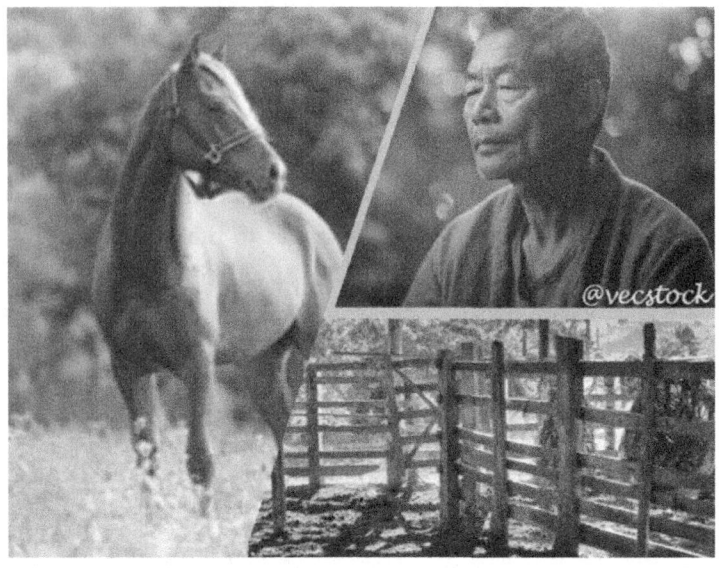

Three days later the horse returned with four other horses and the neighbors clambered over and excitedly exclaimed,

"What good fortune! Excellent fortune! We are so glad!"

The Old Man nodded gently and said,

"We'll see. We'll see."

The next week while his son was breaking one of the new horses, the horse threw him and broke his leg and the neighbors came and said,

"How sad, how bad. We are so sorry for you."

The Old Man nodded gently and said,

"We'll see. We'll see."

The next week soldiers came into the village to take the young men into the army. They left the Old Man's son due to his broken leg. Several weeks later their entire regiment was killed in action.

This man was wise enough to practice open-mindedness and not let himself be carried away into sorrow or elation. He faced each new event with equanimity of soul. I am sure he expressed compassion for his son and his pain. I am sure he had feelings, but he didn't judge in the moment. He had the wisdom to know things are not always what they first appear to be. For you this means this week you say,

"We'll see, we'll see," more of the time.

[1] Julianne Conard channeling Alcazar on equanimity, Stargate Intensive, Thanksgiving 2023. www.thestargateexperienceacademy.com

7

Positivity

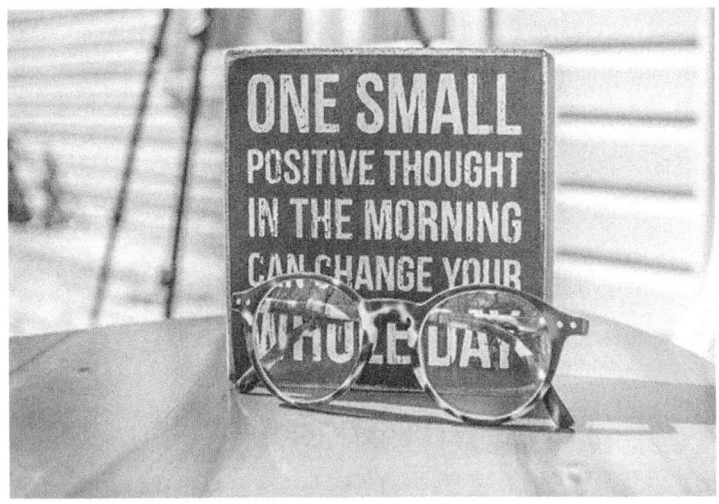

Basic Exercise 4: Positivity –
"To cultivate this soul attitude does not mean to avoid all criticism or to close our eyes to what is bad, false, or inferior. It is not possible to find the bad good and the false true," Rudolph Steiner explains. It does mean attaining an attitude of sympathy

toward all situations, looking for the best possible attributes and keeping an open mind to what could be. It means being humble enough to know you do not know what the ultimate results might be. For example, being laid off or fired. It can be one of the best things, for it can lead to a better position, or starting your own business and being much happier.

"It means responding to what is praiseworthy, seeking out what is to the good, constructive, beautiful in all things and situations. This develops the power to nullify negative influences."

Rudolph Steiner

Here we have an opportunity to STOP the stress locomotive and take the attitude that we don't know everything. That our automatic assumptions may not be valid. Maintaining a positive attitude itself sends out "constructive influences," positive energies. It means taking responsibility for the energies we are putting out and the influences those have on the world around us. It helps us attend to smaller details which can otherwise be overlooked, which can be so helpful in showing us how to turn the situation constructive. To be positive does not mean to be aggressive, only to approach a person or situation in a spirit of constructive interest. It means changing our 'already there' habits. We have learned how to react and we are in the process of reprogramming ourselves to be more constructive.

Just stopping and slowing the process down makes a big difference and gives us new options. Drinking less caffeine can also help this process. Doing exercises in the morning – simple stretches, yoga, Chi Kung or Tai Chi — can set you on a smoother path where you are more able to achieve a state of equanimity. Focus on this for a week. Make note of how this exercise reduces stress for you.

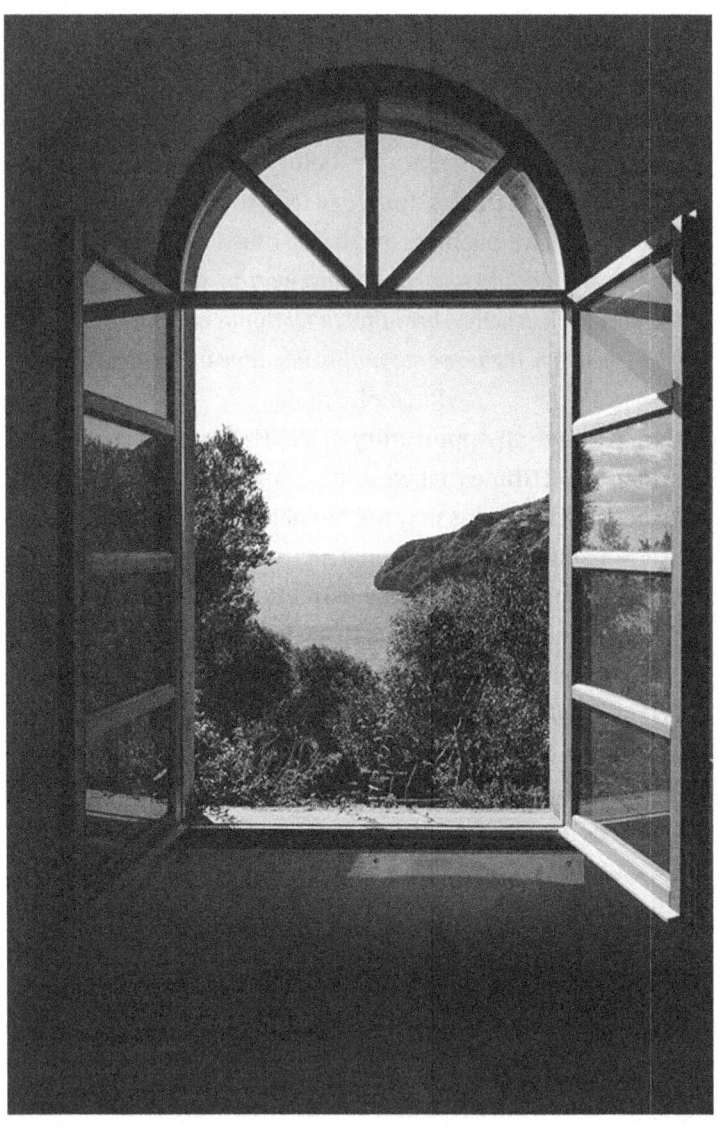

8

Open Mindedness

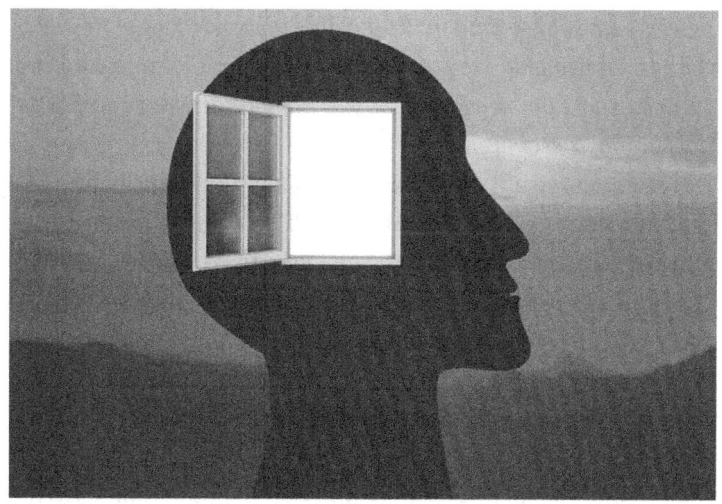

Basic Exercise 5: Open Mindedness – It is very easy today to choose a side and close your mind to other possibilities. Dr. Steiner over a hundred years ago spoke to the need for open-mindedness, today it is even more important. This does not mean to believe everything you see or hear. It is challenging these days to find truth. Many who claim to have it are just selling us a bill of goods that are most likely not good for us. What this exercise is asking is: *"Are we able to be ready at any moment to take in a new idea, a new experience, with total impartiality?"* Written one hundred years ago by Dr. Steiner: *"Life is continually evolving, sometimes at a rapid pace, and we need to see what is for the good and what is detrimental to it; also, how we are to proceed in relating to it. New manifestations of truth must find us ready at any time to receive them. Our thinking and our impulses of will grow more mature as we freely take in, without bias, what is new. While we do not disregard past ideas and experiences, we must be willing to continually experience what is new. We must have faith in the possible contradictions of the old by the new, as being the way of evolution. Therefore, we implant in our consciousness the need never to fail in maintaining an impartial, open mind, free of prejudice."*

It's an exercise. It's an exercise in changing our habits and our outlook. Saying, "It could be..." This is often used in good communication as a way to not engage in arguments with someone of very differing ideas. "Hmmmm, it could be..." leaves room for reflection and processing. After all, remember that the idea of men flying was once considered crazy and it wasn't that long ago as history wends its way through time.

My grandmother was born in 1883 and in 1969 I asked her if she thought the men would land on the moon. She gave her usual harumph and gesture and said,

"Honey, I remember when the first streetlights went in here." She gestured outside deep in the city of Chicago. She proceeded to tell me about the gas lighting men whose job it was to go around and light the streetlights.

"At that time the street was dirt and the method of travel was

horse and buggy. So why not land on the moon?" was her attitude.

I realized in that moment just how much change her generation had endured in the past hundred years and how much has changed since then is enormous.

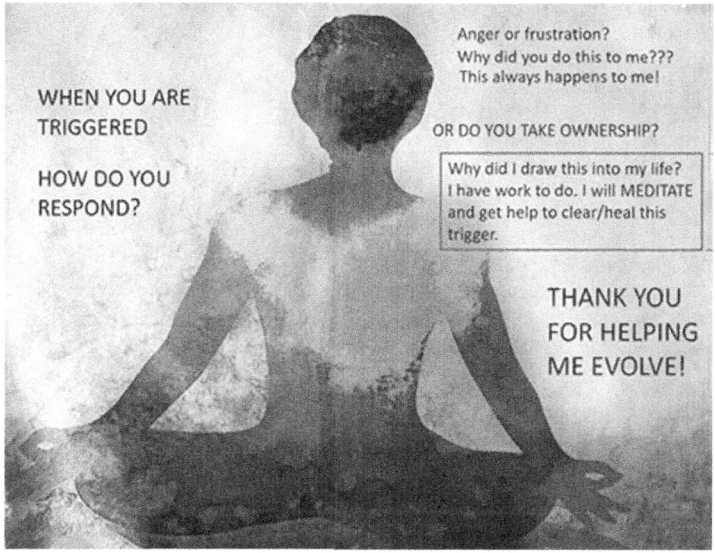

L Marks Photos

A change in your attitude might include changing the blame game. Do you tend to blame your reactions on others' actions? We sometimes learn this in childhood and never grow out of it. As we evolve, we begin to ask,

"What is the trigger in me that needs to be healed?"

Consider working with the outlook that we draw situations to us that help us to heal and grow. They are sometimes quite uncomfortable and when we take that information in, we have an opportunity to grow. This can be using the Open-Mindedness

Exercise to great benefit.

How does this exercise reduce stress in your life?

9

Cycling all Five Basic Exercises

Exercise 6 Cycling - very important - When you have successfully completed one consecutive cycle of 7 days of each of the above five exercises begin now to practice them again but with more frequent interchange. Do them in pairs, one pair each day for a week; another pair the next week, and so on for five weeks.

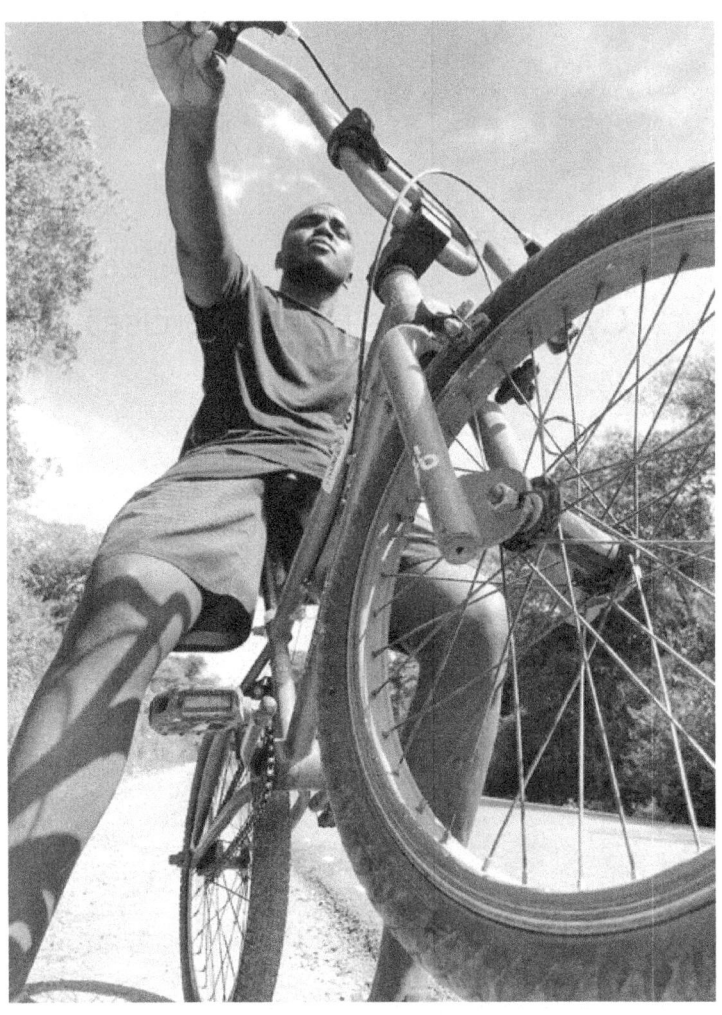

You may also practice one exercise per day for several weeks. You can also do them one month at a time. Great results will eventually become apparent.

"These exercises are suitable for anyone to do who is in earnest about it," said Rudolf Steiner. *"The important point is not to aim*

for any special achievement —such as attaining 'spiritual vision,' 'enlightenment,' or the like -~ but to keep steadily going in the direction one has chosen, regardless of results. Whereas the usual attitude in our material world is to 'go get,' and accomplish, spiritual results come of themselves when we practice steadily. Spiritual qualities, their value, come to us, but only when we are ready to receive them; to bear them." He also said *"When these exercises are conscientiously carried out it will be found that they yield gradually, much more than at first appeared to be in them...Continuity of effort builds the power of control, more can be gained by extending the practice period to two, three or even four weeks. This of course requires more discipline to maintain the longer stretch without a break, but such discipline brings far-reaching rewards. Gradually it develops in the soul firmness, certainty, equilibrium, and that consistency which makes for "character". Therefore, try one month on each exercise if you can sustain it."*

Rudolph Steiner Knowledge of Higher Worlds, ISBN: 088010046X , Steiner Books, 1983

After you have mastered keeping your object or phrase steady, let the object/phrase go and keep a clear mind for 5 minutes. If your mind wanders go back to your object/phrase for a time and then try empty mind again. Once you get the hang of it, you will want to be here for more than 5 minutes.

How has this reduced stress for you?

Rudolph Steiner *Knowledge of Higher Worlds*, ISBN: 088010046X , Steiner Books, 1983

10

Rückshau – Looking Back Exercise

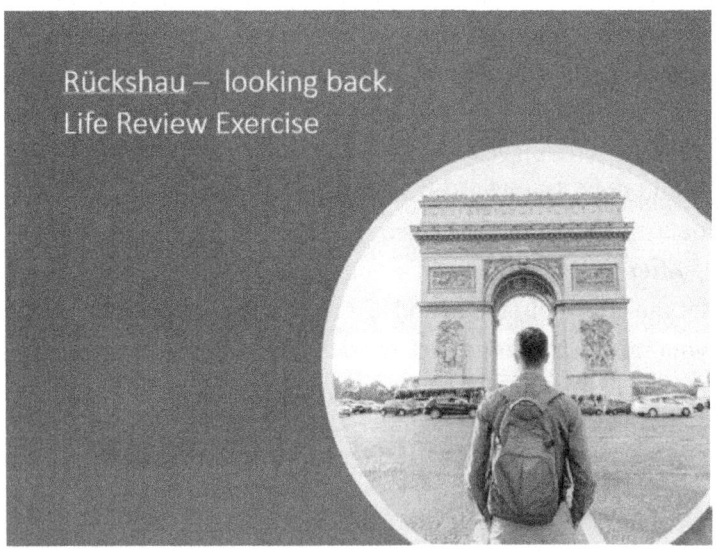

The Rückshau is not part of the five basic exercises, but it is one of Rudolph Steiner's. It is an exercise designed to empty your body, mind and soul in a good way. It is especially helpful when you've had a challenging day or a situation with which you just don't feel at ease. It requires you to sit in quiet meditation focusing your mind (learned through Exercise 1 above). The goal is to run your day backwards from the current moment all the way through until when you first woke this morning. Imagine a movie reel where you can run the reel backward and leave it on the viewing room floor. Imagine you can rewind it at a very fast speed once you gain the skills of doing this exercise. What will happen is that when a part of your day needs to be reviewed it will slow down so that you can see someone else's reaction or something that you missed. Our subconscious (or super conscious) minds often pick up on cues we miss and this exercise gives the super conscious permission to bring to your attention the things you need to know. I've also found this helpful to use after seeing a movie that had a strong impression on me – one that kept getting in the way of my thoughts and concentration. Sitting in meditation and running the movie backward, sometimes several times, seems to clear this and improves my concentration.

Rudolph Steiner said that if you do the Rückshau diligently and regularly, it will save you time during your life review after your physical death. You've probably heard of people with close calls or near-death experiences telling of seeing their life flashing before their eyes. This is the life review process.

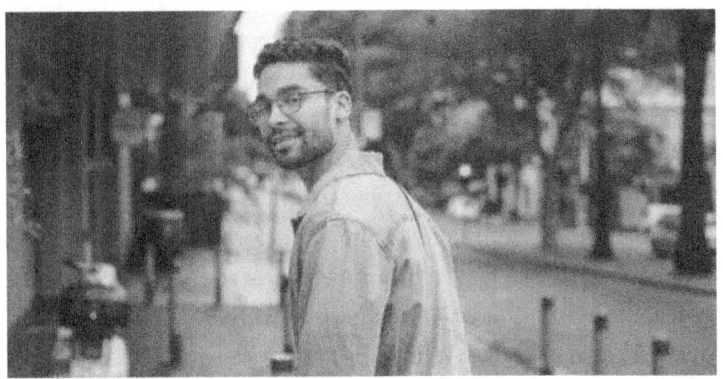

Looking back gives greater freedom to move forward. You can use this while working with the Five Basic Exercises or while you are taking a break from them.

"When I have been running and running, busy, busy, busy, I stop and realize I have not had time to digest/process my experiences, I sit and do the Rückshau sometimes for an entire week! It helps me relax and make space for what's coming next."

Teacher, Chicago, Illinois

11

Physical and Energetic Helpers

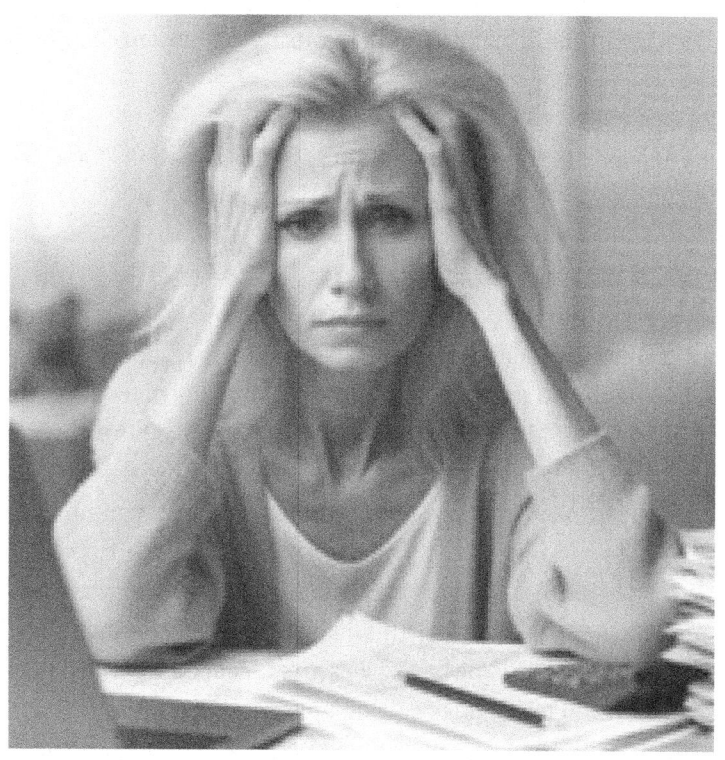

One year, as a young adult while working on my bookkeeping prep for taxes, I realized I was very stressed. My shoulders were up and aching, there was tightness in my chest and abdomen and a general feeling of nerves. I had taken up yoga some years before and started doing the Five Basic Exercises, both of which increased my awareness. Because I had consciously set an intention to change the patterns of stress in my life, I became aware that year of the stress level doing taxes and how unhelpful that response was. I took responsibility and set my intention to learn how to do my taxes without stress. My taxes would be what they would be. My stress would not change the bottom line. I did some deep breathing, grounded and went to my meditation chair with several questions. One was:

"When did I first respond stressfully to this situation?" and the second was,

"Where did I learn to be this way?"

I sat quietly wondering how I had learned this response. After a time of quiet, a memory of my father doing his taxes came up in my mind and I could see I was acting just like him. Several old movie scenes with men reacting badly to financial situations including taxes came up out of remote access in my mind.

Since I had been doing the Five Basic Exercises, I knew what to do next and I was able to break this habit with some conscious effort. I set my intention. The payoff was great. I added some behavior modification techniques setting up rewards for myself when I worked without stress for a given period of time. I used yoga stretching and meditation/relaxation music before sitting down to work on taxes and agreed with myself that I would only work on taxes as long as I could remain calm. In the beginning I only managed 5 to 10 minutes without stress even after considerable yoga and relaxation music. Once stress started, I returned to yoga or went for a walk. I will admit the first year I got more yoga than taxes done. I had to file for an extension but it was worth it. Each year it got better and within a few years I could do taxes stress free. That has given me many years of stress-free tax times. This is a good example of situation specific stress.

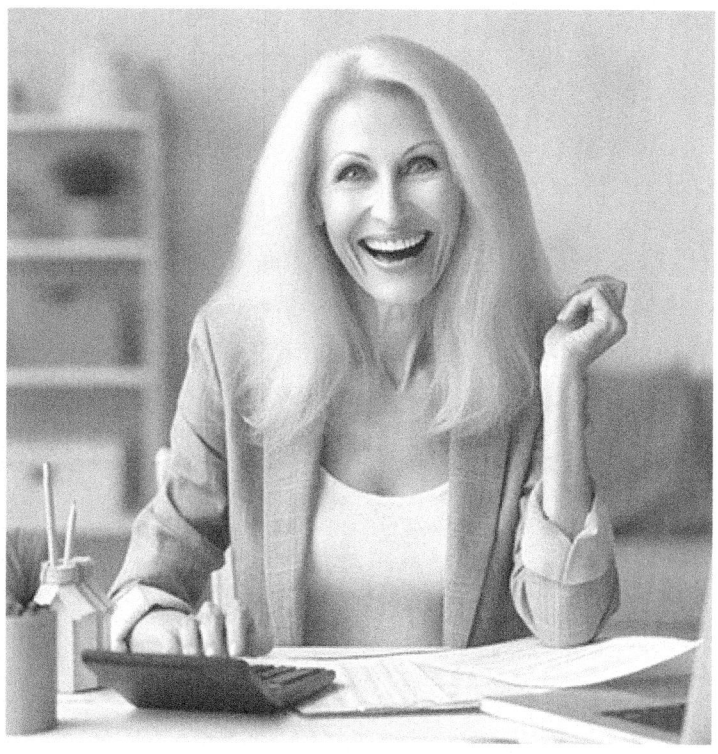

Tai Chi or Chi Kung – are both physical and energetic practices which will greatly enhance your life with little effort. Look on YouTube to start to find an instructor you like and begin with a short morning exercise and observe the results in your life. This is no monetary cost. Next you might want to try adding an evening routine. I find in my life investing 10 to 15 minutes a day in either or both of these disciplines pays back the time saved during the day and quality of sleep during the night. Try and see for yourself.

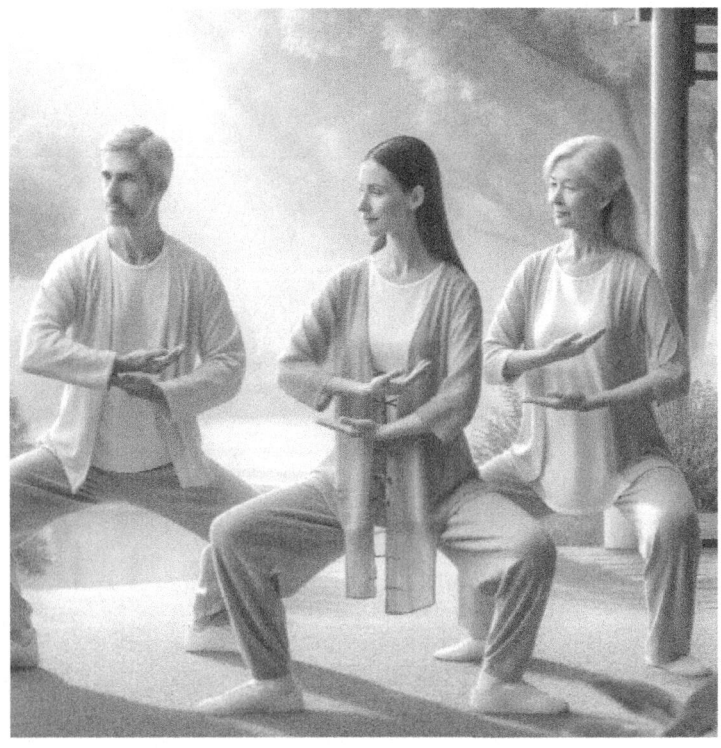

Yoga does not have to be extreme. Again, start with YouTube and see who you like as an instructor and what style you like. There are many to choose from. I rather like the Yoga flow routines with good warmups and cool downs with deeper stretches. Yoga Rebel is an app you can purchase. It provides a variety of yoga routines with an emphasis on Yoga Flow.

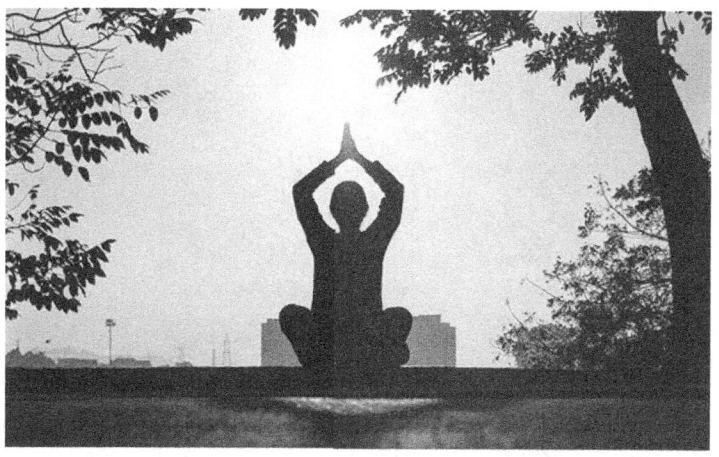

Walk – when things get stressful, take a walk. If the weather allows, go outside, if not go to a mall or gym where you can walk or run.

THE TRUTH ABOUT STRESS

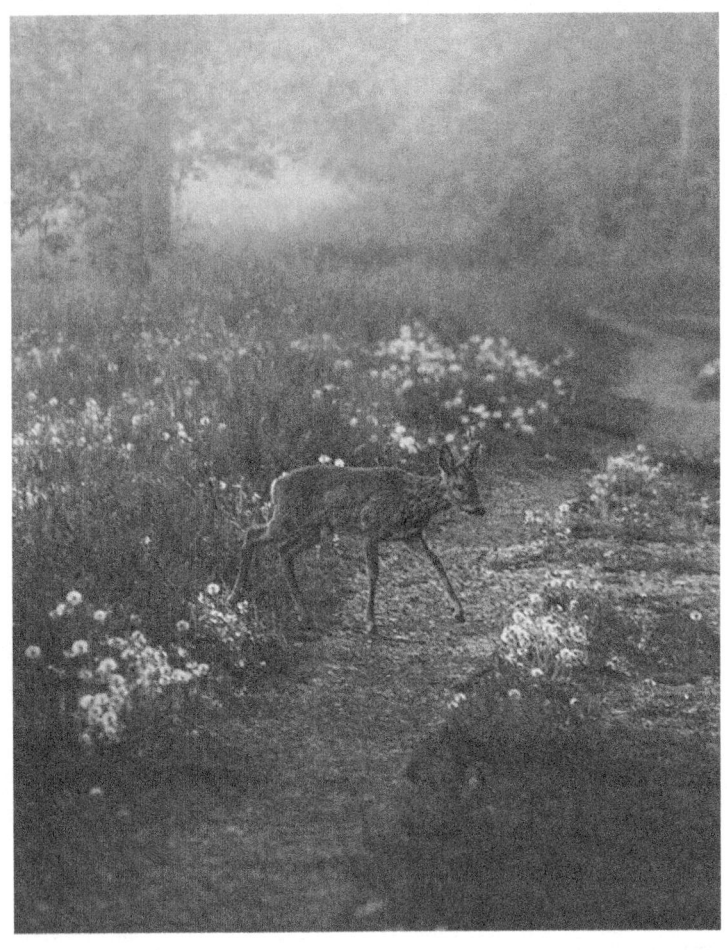

12

Conclusion and Continuance

CONCLUSION AND CONTINUANCE

Stress is mostly within your control and to find this control the exercises presented in this book provide a platform for you to practice and observe how they change your life. All that's left is for you to do them and repeat them. They have worked for many people, I'm confident they will work for you too.

Think about your life after doing these exercises.

What percent of the time do you feel stressed now? 1-100 _____

What level of stress do you experience now? 1-100 _____.

Enter these figures in your Journal with the date and compare them to those you first recorded (your baseline). Keep going and you will see more progress. Every time you complete a round of these exercises, record your stress level and date it so you can keep track of your progress.

Hoping for happy stress-free times ahead for you.

I sincerely hope you enjoyed this book and that you will find greater freedom from stress in your life as a result. If you did, I would greatly appreciate it if you would take a few minutes to write a **quick review on Amazon or whatever platform you purchased it from**. That means so much.

You can also join a class. The Class I teach is a webinar format and takes the ideas of this book, expands on them and provides a place to practice them in a supportive community where you will have accountability and a place to have your questions answered. Working with a group creates a larger energetic and can provide a supercharge to your work. It will also give you a supportive community to discuss issues around the exercises and explore solutions. .

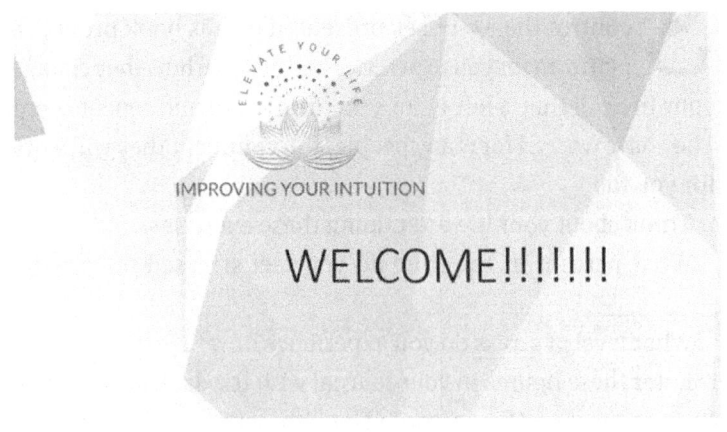

IMPROVING YOUR INTUITION WEBINARS from Body, Soul & Angels provide this support. If you are interested in attending a Webinar, please visit: www.Bodysoulandangels.com/Improvving

yourituition and sign up to receive news about the next series of classes. You can also email Lyneahmarks@bodysoulandangels.com for more information. Looking forward to working with you to help you deepen your connection with yourself and your calm nature.

What students have said about this Webinar:

"An awakening experience. This class gives you tools that you can continue to use in everyday life to help strengthen your abilities. I highly recommend anyone wanting to be more in tune with their higher selves and their happiness to take this class."
  Shannon Trudeau, LMBT, North Carolina

> "Lyneah's classes have had a profound effect on my life in many ways. I have sharpened my intuitive skills greatly and have even repeated classes experiencing new growth each time. I love how it enhances my life and I feel I have advanced on my true path as a result."   Allysha Bounds, Lawrenceville, GA

"Lyneah's class on "Improving Your Intuition" provides the tools that I think are latent in everyone and ready to be used but often aren't. It is a process and the class builds week to week. If you miss a class, it is available as a video replay the next day to get your simple, engaging assignment for the next week. Certainly, everyone will have a different result in their particular life but I did notice subtle changes in my life where instead of events, positive or negative, being done to me, now were being done for me. Doors closed for several years of work, opened with little further effort on my part. I'll be one of the veterans from this class to sign up for it again

to continue this process of learning. This class on intuition which involved meeting with the other students in real time on Zoom was that valuable to me."

Jim McKelvey, Professional Photographer and Author, North Carolina

"The wealth of knowledge brought together through Lyneah's many years of practice and the diversity of tools and techniques, the breadth of knowledge among the participants and the subjects covered created an exponential learning experience. It was amazing how the information and connections flowed. I am truly grateful for the remembrance of the deeply embedded knowledge that came forth and the way in which we applied it into working projects. Utilizing the tools and tips presented by Lyneah will greatly complement your current toolbox."

April P, Florida

"Lyneah's classes have had a profound and very positive effect on my word view. Not only are the abilities presented and honed in her class of immediate value, — the real-life confirmations are beyond magical. I came as a curious student and left as a passionate and well-equipped advocate and guardian for our beloved Gaia."

Steven Sidhartha Fischer, California

13

Bonus Meditation

Interestingly, Michael is the only archangel mentioned in most of the religions around the world. In this verse, Michael is called upon for his strength and courage in challenging times. Many, regardless of religion or lack of religion, have found help in these verses said morning and night. Give them an open-minded try and see what happens. Skeptical? That's great! Skeptics are not closed-minded. Skeptics say: "We'll see, We'll see," and work with things with an open mind and observe carefully.*

1. FOR THIS MICHAELIC AGE Rudolph Steiner

We must eradicate from the soul all fear and terror of what comes toward man out of the future. We must acquire serenity in all feelings and sensations about the future. We must look forward, with absolute equanimity, to everything that may come and we must think only that whatever comes is given to us by a world direction full of wisdom. It is part of what we must learn in this age; namely to live out of pure trust, without any security in existence, trust in the ever-present help of the spiritual world. Truly, nothing else will do, if our courage is not to fail us. Let us seek the awakening from within ourselves, every morning and every evening.

1. **MORNING**
2. **O, Michael, under Your protection I place myself, with Your guidance I connect myself, wholeheartedly,**

So that this day may become an image of your destiny-ordering Will.

1. **EVENING**
2. **I carry my sorrow into the setting sun, place all my worries into her radiating womb,**

Purified in love, transformed in light, they return as helping thoughts, as strength for self-sacrificing deeds.

This verse has been invested with much energy over many years and has a powerful essence of its own. When you work with this verse:

1. memorize the verses.
2. recite the verses daily morning and evening.
3. set an intention to connect with the essence of the verse.
4. continue reciting it until you connect with the essence.
5. once you experience the essence, you can instantly connect with the it and you've done the meditation. It takes only

a millisecond. It's an interesting experience and requires patience and persistence to achieve.

14

Journal

JOURNAL

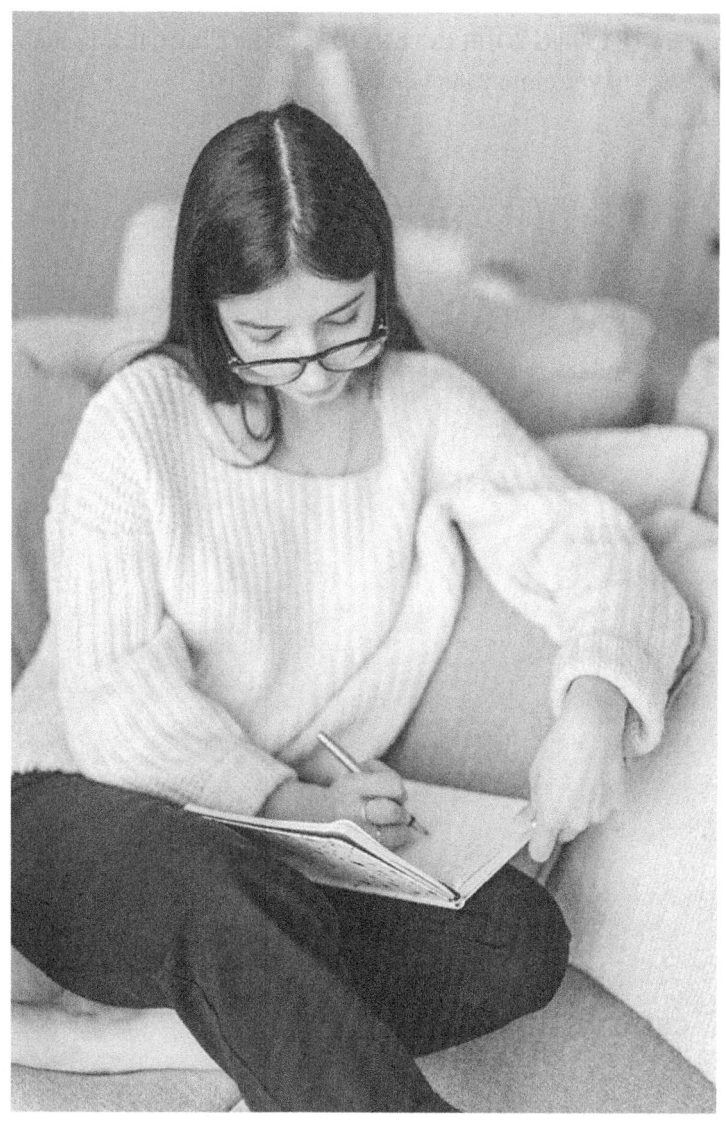

SETTING YOUR INTENTION: make a formal statement of your intention here:

CURRENT STRESS %: _____
CURRENT STRESS LEVEL: _____

TO DO'S:

Date Item Done

Thanks for reading. Thanks for trying the exercises.
Thanks for growing.
Thanks for reducing stress and increasing character.
WWW.BODYSOULANDANGELS.COM

15

Notes/Observations

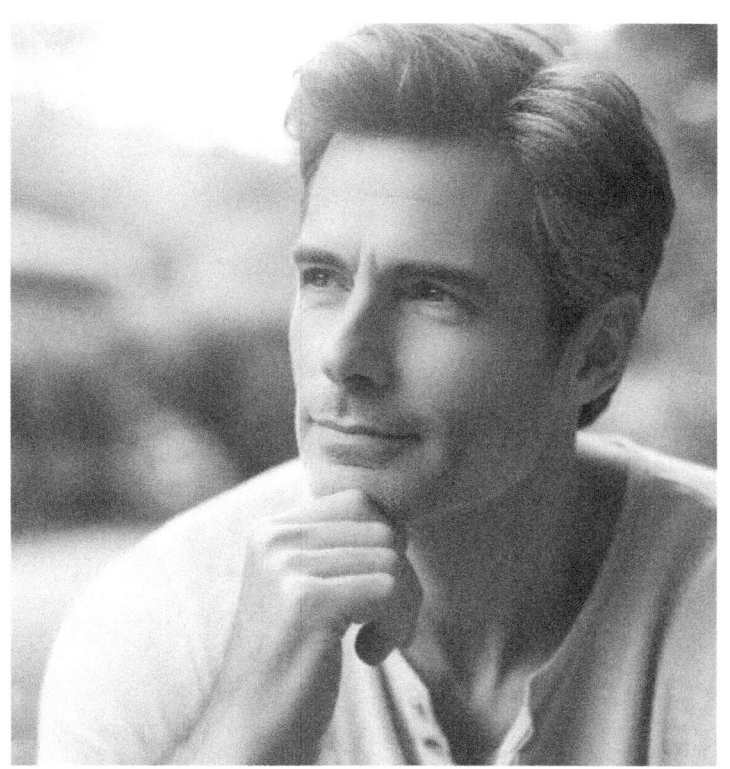

DATE OBSERVATION COMMENT QUESTION

Also by Lyneah Marks

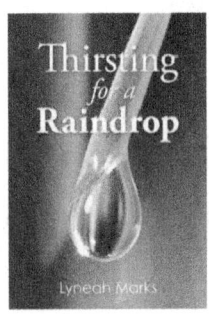

Thirsting for a Raindrop

They say the truth is stranger than fiction. You hold proof in your hands. A childhood filled with extraordinary experiences, an extended visit to the Center for Rehabilitation of the Over-Educated, and the challenges of loss and recovery weave together to form a fascinating tapestry of inspiration and encouragement. If you want help navigating life's challenges, this book is the inspiration you need to transform the dark times to light.

"An inspiring and heroic journey of manifestation that teaches us everything is possible if we believe. This is the best thing I've read in a long time. My eyes were burning and I had to read more." Fonda Joyce, former business manager for Jean Houston and assistant to Chet Huntley

"Thirsting for a Raindrop is so fascinating; I could not put it down. Woven with magic and mystery. Lyneah Marks' memoir is a brilliantly written book that speaks to one woman's strength along with her capacity to surrender to Spirit. Lyneah's life has been a profound journey of challenges and miracles with her remarkable gifts as an intuitive and healer. Read this book and be very inspired!"

Mare Cromwell, award winning author of The Great Mother Bible.

THIRSTING FOR JOY

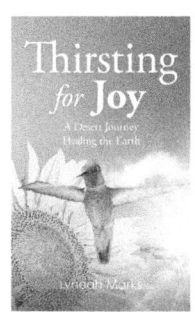

This book is an adventure of transformation on so many levels. I loved it and can't wait to travel further with Lyneah's amazing life. Fonda Joyce, retired manager for Jean Houston

"I thoroughly enjoyed every page and look forward to more. It is so relatable yet gives me a nudge onto the path." Tara

"Lyneah has had so many experiences and every time I read one, it is very edifying to my journey as I can see her magic and her struggles reflected in my own. It is very comforting, supportive and revealing. Thank you Lyneah for this treasure... and it IS a treasure. I am honored to know you."Zephyr (Cheryl) Osborn

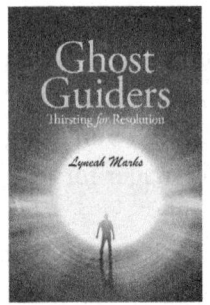
GHOST GUIDERS

What comes to mind when you hear the word *ghost*? Something terrible that can hurt you? Aunt Bessie? *Casper the Friendly Ghost*? *Ghostbusters*? Do you have things that go bump in the night? What to do? This book could help.

Lyneah has seen ghosts since early childhood. Some so sad it sparked a heart desire for helping them. This book tells real ghost stories and explains what was done to help.

Whether you love ghost stories or have a desire to help them, you will find this book fascinating.

"I have worked with Lyneah for about 16 years. She has taught me that the metaphysical is not something to be afraid of, just looked at with understanding, love, and equanimity of soul. Lyneah guides us through the processes. ***I highly recommend this book to anyone interested in the spirit world.****"*

- Allysha Bounds, client of more than 16 years

"Lyneah's books always provide me with unexpected insights and clarity through her stories and joyful attitude while helping others. Her sessions and guidance are always spot on. I hope you enjoy them as much as I have. "

Julie Collins, MS, CHC, LMT, NASM-CPT, CES, NPTI, Peak Wellness and Feng Shui

Lyneah Marks, MA, Soul Integration Therapist, Stargate Facilitator, intuitive and inspired teacher of Earth Healing and Guiding Ghosts forward, lives in Mt Shasta, CA. In this, her third book, she shares her passion for aiding both the humans who are visited by ghosts and the ghosts themselves. To learn more visit www.BodySoulandAngels.com

Made in the USA
Coppell, TX
25 June 2024